# Baby Names

*Enjoy Finding The Perfect Name For Your Baby Through The Most Complete And Simple Baby Name Guide With Special Meanings*

# Table of Contents

Introduction ..................................................................... 3
Chapter 1: Choosing the Perfect Name for Your Baby ............ 4
Chapter 2: Celebrity Baby Names ......................................... 9
Chapter 3: Impression Specific Names ................................ 19
Chapter 4: Biblical Baby Names .......................................... 25
Chapter 5: Unique Baby Names ........................................... 33
Chapter 6: Top 100 Baby Names ......................................... 40
Chapter 7: Top Baby Names of 2018 .................................... 50
Chapter 8: Traditional Baby Names ..................................... 56
Chapter 9: Additional Baby Names A-Z .............................. 62
Conclusion ......................................................................... 68

# Introduction

Congratulations on purchasing *Baby Names* and congratulations on your impending bundle of joy. While having a baby is undeniably a joyous occasion, there are a million things that need to be taken care of before the big day, making the difficulties inherent in choosing a new baby name even more troublesome to manage.

Luckily, the following chapters will discuss everything you need to keep in mind when it comes to choosing the right baby name, while also giving you a laundry list of names in a wide variety of categories. You will find a list of the latest celebrity baby names, so you know what to choose, or what to avoid, based on your personal preference. Next you will find a list of names that have become associated with specific traits, such as strength or intelligence to steer your child in a specific direction. You will then find a chapter on Biblical names, before one on unique baby names, depending on which direction you want to go based on your beliefs.

From there you will find the list of the 100 most popular baby names, as well as the list of the most popular names that experts will expect to see in 2018. You will then find a list of traditional baby names as well as a long list of names that don't easily fit into any of the other categories.

Every effort was made to ensure this book is full of as much useful information as possible, please enjoy!

# Chapter 1: Choosing the Perfect Name for Your Baby

If you are already feeling some anxiety when it comes to choosing the perfect name for your child, don't worry this is perfectly natural. After all, you need to pick something that is going to be with your child for their entire life which is, to put it mildly, a lot of pressure. Furthermore, you will likely hear input, wanted or not, from virtually everyone who finds out you are having a baby which means all the noise can start to build up and make it easy for everything to feel overwhelming. Keep the following in mind to ensure you pick the best name possible.

*Consider the sound of the name:* While it can be easy to like a name on paper, it is equally important to ensure that you say the name allowed plenty of times before you make your decision; after all, you are going to be hearing it quite often which means that choosing the right sounds is key. It is important to choose a name that sounds pleasant to the ear, as those that are harsh often have negative connotations attached. Likewise, make sure to say it in conjunction with your last name which is how your child will be using it much of the time. Catching something early that sounds odd, rhymey, or like a pun can certainly save your child grief later in life and is certainly worth considering as well. While you might like the sound of a rhyming or pun name now, rest assured that the joke will wear off long before other people get tired of it.

Additionally, you will want to consider your feelings on if you like a longer first name when compared to the last name, vice versa, or two names of equal length. Furthermore, some people believe that having the first name end with a vowel while the last name also starts with a vowel can make it easy for the names to bleed together.

# Baby Names

*Unique, but not too unique:* While no one wants to have a child, who will ultimately end up being one of four or more children in the same class with the same name, it is important to not over-correct too far in the opposite direction either. While a unique name can certainly set your child apart while also giving them a name with some real meaning to it, it is important to carefully consider any unique names before committing to them entirely. The reason for this is because it is extremely easy for unique names to go overboard on their uniqueness, leading to a lifetime of extra hassle for your child.

As such, when you choose a unique name, the first thing you are going to want to do is to ensure that it is as easy to spell as possible. If you can find a unique name that is spelled like it sounds, great, otherwise keep things as simple as possible. Remember, your child is likely going to be spelling their name throughout school, every time they are on the phone with a customer service representative, every time they put their name in at a restaurant, the list goes on and on. Taking the extra time to ensure this process is as smooth as possible is literally going to save them hundreds of hours over their lifetime and makes choosing a basic spelling one of the most crucial parts of considering unique names.

If you like the idea of a more common name, but still feel the desire to mix things up, then a unique spelling might be a viable option. When considering alternate spellings, however, it is important to not get too out of hand. For example, double Es instead of a Y is a popular naming these days, but it could easily get out of hand and lead to lengthy conversations about the spelling of the name in moments when your child just wants to get on with whatever it is they are doing.

Furthermore, above all else when it comes to naming conventions, form should never supersede function. Put another way, your unique spelling should never get so unique that people can't determine how the name is pronounced just by reading it. No one likes to have to speak up with a correction to their name and adding too many spelling flourishes to the name is essentially ensuring your child is going to have to do that regularly for their entire life.

*Understand the significance:* While it can be easy to pick names based simply on the way they sound or because they have been passed down through your family for generations, it is important to always consider the meaning of your favorite names as well, as the benefits of doing so are two-fold. First, you may find that your favorite or family names have a greater meaning than you would have ever expected. For example, the name Ingrid might not be on your list until you learn that it mean's hero's daughter which could make it the perfect way to honor military service in your family.

*Don't forget about the initials:* While your child's initials won't come up today as much as they might have in the past, it is still worth consider. For example, if your last name is Thomas then naming your daughter Zara Ilene might lead to some easily avoidable trouble in school. Again, if you come up with the perfect name and the only thing standing in your way is the initials, then you will need to consider the pros and cons of going with what you have chosen or of going in an alternate direction instead.

*Pick a name for all seasons:* While a name like Bunny, Lucky, or Rusty might seem to fit your baby perfectly, it is important to keep in mind that the name is going to have to travel with them throughout their lives as well. While this might be a cute choice for a three-year-old, when they are interviewing for jobs or going on dates in their 30s then it might seem far less so. As a general rule, it is better to choose a name that will serve the child as an adult and then choose a nickname that is more suited to a child. Richard, for example, is great for Richie the child as well. This gives the child the opportunity to shed the childish version of their name or keep it if it ends up suiting their personality.

*Use the middle name to come to agreements:* It is perfectly natural to have close friends and family members pressuring you to choose a name for your baby based on heritage, tradition, that bet you lost in college, whatever it may be. A great way to satisfy these people, if it is important to you to do so, while still choosing a name that you like and believe the child can live with, is to give over the middle name slot to the sentimental name while still ensuring that your name has top billing. You can also use the sentimental name as the primary name while using the middle name as the name the child commonly goes by. While this is somewhat cumbersome, it is a common enough naming convention that your child won't have to explain it nearly as often as say, a name with an odd pronunciation based on the spelling.

**Dealing with naming disagreements**
While pregnancy can certainly bring partners together, the process of choosing the name of your future child has just as much chance of driving them apart as well. Consider the following tips to help you and your significant other come to an amiable agreement from both sides.

*Be sure to listen:* When we argue, it is easy to get into the mindset where we are focusing more on how to defend our own argument than what the other person actually has to say. Needless to say, this is a great way to start a fight and a bad way to make any progress when it comes to choosing a baby name that everyone is happy with. As such, if you find yourself fighting with your significant other then the best place to start is by trying to actively listen to the other person.

Feeling heard naturally decreases tension among all parties, making them more amiable to compromise. To show that you are listening, use the things they are saying in your responses, without making it sound as though you are trying to make a counterpoint. Instead, strive to show that you understand what the other person is saying, even if you disagree with the crux of their argument. This will have the benefit of making it easier for you to come up with ideas that can work as reasonable compromises for both parties.

*Retain perspective:* While deciding on the name of your future child can seem like a very personal, very important fact in the moment, the truth of the matter is that there are far more important considerations about the future of the child than what to call them. Nevertheless, during the conversation about the name it is only natural that emotions run high, especially if one party's favorite name is dismissed out of hand. While this sort of blanket rejection can feel like a personal attack, it is important to instead remember that this is not the case. Choosing a baby name isn't a competition it should be a mutual process that is about coming to an agreement about what is best for the child. Check your ego and your emotions at the door and you will find that the process proceeds much more smoothly.

**Baby name test**
For the following test, you are going to want to wait until you have looked through all the names provided so that you can come up with the best results possible. Once you and your significant other have both picked out your top five names, you will then want to rate the other person's in the following categories.
- Spelling
- Pronunciation
- Sound
- Last Name
- Gender ID
- Nicknames
- Popularity
- Uniqueness
- First Impression
- Namesakes
- Initials
- Meaning

For each one of these categories you are going to want give the name **1** point if you feel positive about that name for that specific category, **0** points if you feel neutral about it and **-1** point if you feel the name does not stand up well in that category. The name with the most points will make your decision. When you come across specific aspects of a given name that you don't like, be sure to make note of specifically what about the name strikes you the wrong way as this will help you talk about it rationally with your partner at a later time.

Once you have tallied up your points, it should then be much easier for you to rate the names that your partner has chosen that you like, and the ones you can't stand. Remember, choosing a baby name is all about give and take, and using the results of this list should at least give you both some common ground to start from.

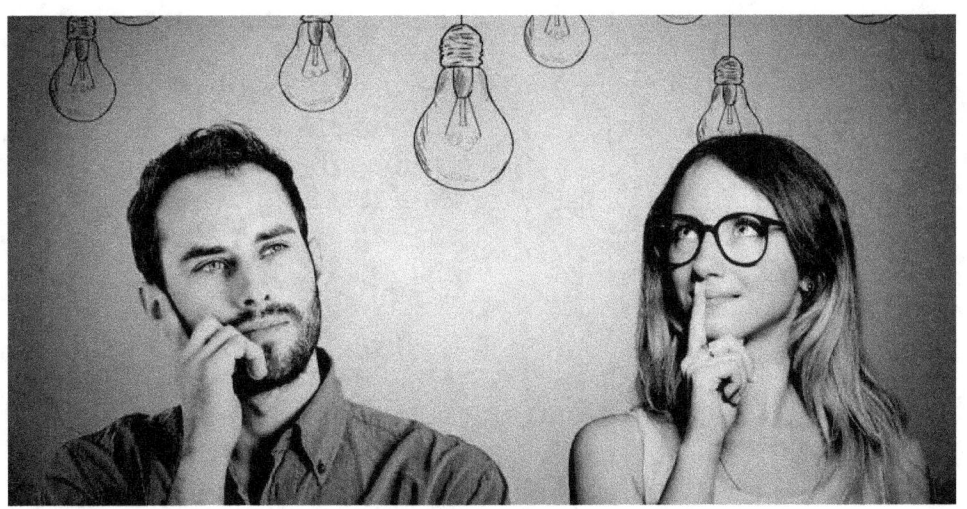

# Chapter 2: Celebrity Girl Names

## Celebrity girl names

Ada James (Thomas Rhett and Lauren Akins)
Alba (Adam Clayton and Mariana Teixeira De Carvalho)
Alexis Kerry (Josh Altman and Heather Bilyeu Altman)
Alexis Olympia (Serena Williams and Alexis Ohanian)
Alice Rose (and twin sister Gracie Jane) (Ronnie Wood and Sally Wood)
Amada Lee (Eva Mendes and Ryan Gosling)
Amalia (Natalie Portman and Benjamin Millepied)
Arrow Rhodes (and twin brother Zeppelin Bram) (Jensen Ackles and Danneel Harris)
Atlee Bay (Bristol Palin and Dakota Meyer)
August (Mark Zuckerberg and Priscilla Chan)
Bari Najma (Mahershala Ali and Amatus Sami-Karim)
Batel Lu (Jenna Jameson and Lior Bitton)
Bella Raine (Derek and Hannah Jeter)
Bennett Alejandra (Briga Heelan and Rene Gube)
Bianka Bella (Kobe Bryant and Vanessa Bryant)
Birdie Joe (Brie Bella and Daniel Bryan)
Bodhi Soleil (Nikki Reed and Iam Somerhalder)
Bowie Rose (Dane DeHaan and Anna Wood)
Calliope Maeve (Felicia Day)
Caroline (Charles and Lizzy Shaffer)
Caroline (Megan Boone and Dan Estabrook)
Charlie (Alona Tal and Marcos Ferraez)
Clara Elizabeth (Anna Chlumsky and Shaun So)
Cleo James (Nev Schulman and Laura Perlongo)
Coco Rae (and twin sister Gia James) (Dan Reynolds and Aja Volkman)
Daisy Alice Winnie (Saffron Burrows and Alison Balian)
Daisy Josephine (Olivia Wilde and Jason Sudeikis)
Dolly Grace (Kimberly and Stephen Schlapman)
Dream Renée (Blac Chyna and Rob Kardashian)
Dusty Rose (Adam Levine and Behati Prinsloo)

# Baby Names

Ella (and twin brother Alexander) (George and Amal Clooney)
Ella Grace (Keshia Knight Pulliam and Ed Hartwell)
Ella Loren (Tika Sumpter and Nicholas James)
Ella Rose (Laura Benanti and Patrick Brown)
Elle (Bar Refaeli and Adi Ezra)
Emery Farryn (Josh Abbott and Taylor Parnell)
Emilia (James Van Der Beek and Kimberly Van Der Beek)
Emily (Sutton Foster and Ted Griffin)
Ensley Jolie (Jenelle Evans and David Eason)
Esme Olivia (Eric Christian Olsen and Sarah Wright Olsen)
Essex Reese (J.P. and Ashley Herbert Rosenbaum)
Estere (and twin sister Stelle) (Madonna)
Eva Maria Dos Santos (and twin brother Mateo Ronaldo) (Cristiano Ronaldo)
Evangeline (Dylan Farrow and Dana Silver)
Ever Lee Wilde (Nicholas Gonzalez and Kelsey Crane-Gonzalez)
Flora (Carter Oosterhouse and Amy Smart)
Florence May (Candice Accola and Joe King)
Frances ("Frankie") (Sarah Chalke and Jamie Afifi)
Frances Laiz Setta Schenkkan (Morena Baccarin and Ben McKenzie)
Freya (Jake and Stephanie McLaughlin)
Georgia (Morgan Olsen Smith and Joel Smith)
Georgia Grace (Jenni Pulos and Dr. Jonathan Nassos)
Gia James (and twin sister Coco Rae) (Dan Reynolds and Aja Volkman)
Gloria (Robert Griffin and Grete Sadeiko)
Gracie Jane (and twin sister Alice Rose) (Ronnie Wood and Sally Wood)
Haley Joy (Hoda Kotb)
Hayden (Camilla Luddington and Matthew Alan)
Heiress Diana (Tameka "Tiny" Harris and Clifford "T.I." Harris)
Holland Rose Madeleine (Erica Rose and Galen Gentry)
Ines (Blake Lively and Ryan Reynolds)
Iris May (Eddie Redmayne and Hannah Bagshawe)
Izzy Oona (Eddie Murphy and Paige Butcher)

# Baby Names

Jonelle (Jimy and Stacey DeMartini)
Jordana Nicole (Zachery Ty Bryan and Carly Bryan)
Josephine Kate (Jessica Capshaw and Christopher Gavigan)
Julia Mimi Bella (Lacey Chabert and David Nehdar)
Justice (Nate Parker and Sarah Di Santo Madeline)
Kirra Max (Audrina Patridge and Corey Bohan)
Lea De Seine (Bradley Cooper and Irina Shayk)
Leia Josephine (Edyta Sliwinska and Alec Mazo)
Lily Grace Victoria (Nicholai Olivia "Nicky" Hilton Rothschild and James Amschel Rothschild)
Liv (Bar Refaeli and Adi Ezra)
Louise (Marion Cotillard and Guillaume Canet)
Love Lily (Preston Brust and Kristen Brust)
Lucille Ruby (Leslie Odom Jr and Nicolette Robinson)
Lula Rose (Liv Tyler and David Gardner)
Luna Simone Stephens (John Legend and Chrissy Teigen)
Lyla Isabela (April Hernandez-Castillo and Jose Castillo)
Lyric Dean (AJ and Rochelle McLean)
Mabel (Russell Brand and Laura Gallagher)
Madilyn Jane (Jonny Fairplay and Caryn Finkbeiner)
Marchesa Anna (Lauren Manzo and Vito Scalia)
Marlow Alice (Amber Tamblyn and David Cross)
Mary Lucille Diana (Zac Hanson and Kate Hanson)
Maya (Gal Gadot and Yaron Versano)
Milena (Ben Cohen and Kristina Rihanoff)
Millie (Colin and Helen O'Donoghue)
Millie June (Curtis and Myranda Rempel)
Molly Sullivan (Ali Fedotowksy and Kevin Manno)
Nixie Barbara (Chad Lowe and Kim Painter)
Odette Elliot (Jared Padalecki and Genevieve Cortese)
Olivia (Kellie Martin and Keith Christian)
Onyx Solace (Alanis Morissette and Mario Treadway)
Payton June (Ike Barinholtz and Erica Hanson)
Pippa Jean (Lindsay Sloane and Dar Rollins)

# Baby Names

Presley Bowie (Jackson Rathbone and Sheila Hafsadi)
Rainey Ryan (Randy and Chelsea Rogers)
Ray (Lisa Ling and Paul Song)
Rayni Bell (Stephen Barker Liles and Jenna Kennedy)
Remi McKenna (Chris Lucas and Kaitlyn Lucas)
Robbie (Rob Schneider and Patricia Schneider)
Rose Elizabeth (Kris Allen and Katy Allen)
Rowan Louise (Mikey Way and Kristin Colby Way)
Rumi (and twin brother Sir) (Beyonce and Jay-Z)
Sailor Stevie (Joanna Garcia Swisher and Nick Swisher)
Sally James (Audra McDonald and Will Swenson)
Scarlett Heleena (Devon Sawa and Dawni Sawa)
Serafina Simone (Sebastian and Lana Maniscalco)
Shane (Erika Christensen and Cole Maness)
Sienna (Poppy Harlow and Sinisa Babcic)
Sienna Princess (Ciara and Russell Wilson)
Sovereign Dior Cambella (Cam Newton and Kia Proctor)
Stella Star (Briana DeJesus and Luis)
Stelle (and twin sister Estere) (Madonna)
Trixie Grace (Emma and Mathew James "Matt" Willis)
Trulee Nanette (Lee Brice and Sara Reeveley)
Valentina Angelina (Kevin Jonas and Danielle Jonas)
Vera Audrey (Emilie de Ravin and Eric Bilitch)
Violet (Emily Blunt and John Krasinski)
Wilder Grace (Alison Pill and Joshua Leonard)
Willow May (Shayne Ward and Sophie Austin)
Winner (Nya Lee)
Wisdom (Kel Mitchell and Asia Lee)
Zoe Dylan (Thomas Ian Nicholas and Colette "DJ Colette" Marino)
Zyla Moon Oluwakemi (Wale Jourdan and Claudia "Chloé" Alexis Jourdan)

**Celebrity boy names**

Ace Thomas (Spike Mendelsohn and Cody Mendelsohn)
Aidan (Chelsea Clinton and Marc Mezvinsky)
Albert (AJ Calloway and Dionne Walker)
Alexander (and twin sister Ella) (George and Amal Clooney)
Alexander Erik Hubertus Bertil (Princess Sofia of Sweden and Prince Carl Philip)
Anacã (Candice Swanepoel and Hermann Nicoli)
Arlo Gale (Holly Williams and Chris Coleman)
Asahd (Khaled Mohamed Khaled "DJ Khaled" and Nicole Tuck)
Ashe Olsen (Seth Meyers and Alexi Meyers)
Asher James (Shay Mooney and Hannah Billingsley)
Asher Wrigley (Desiree Hartsock Siegfried and Chris Siegfried)
Auden James Ellis (Kelsey Grammer and Kayte Grammer)
Augustus Alexis (David and Christina Arquette)
Axel James (Caleb Brush and Maddie Brown)
Axton Joseph (Mia Tyler and Dan Halen)
Bear (Liam Payne and Cheryl Cole)
Beau Dean (Tori Spelling and Dean McDermott)
Beau Rush (Virginia Williams and Bradford Bricken)
Benjamin (Tyler Ritter and Leila Parma)
Bluey (Sam Branson and Isabella Calthorpe)
Bodhi Burton (Burt Jenner and Valerie Pitalo)
Boomer Robert (Michael Phelps and Nicole Johnson)
Bowen Michael (Michael Stagliano and Emily Tuchscherer)
Bowie Juniper (Tess Holliday and Nick Holliday)
Brooks Hartman (Ashley Salter and Austin Brannen)
Caben-Albi George (Stephanie Davis and Jeremy McConnell)
Caiden Zane (Ryan Lochte and Kayla Rae Reed)
Caleb Kelechi (Kerry Washington and Nnamdi Asomugha)
Carter Davis (Danielle Harris and David Gross)
Carter Stone (and twin brother Cash Steven)

# Baby Names

("Robbie E" Strauss and Tara Strauss)
Cash Steven (and twin brother Carter Stone) ("Robbie E" Strauss and Tara Strauss)
Cayson Jack (Melissa Rycroft and Tye Strickland)
Charles Max (Savannah Guthrie and Mike Feldman)
Charlie (James Wolk and Elizabeth Jae Byrd)
Charlie Wolf (Zooey Deschanel and Jacob Pechenik)
Christian Scott (Scott MacIntyre and Christina MacIntyre)
Conor Jack (Conor McGregor and Dee Devlin)
Cruz Achille (Mara Schiavocampo and Tommie Porter)
Cypress Night (Jack Huston and Shannan Click)
Daren O.C. ("Doc") (Shanola Hampton and Daren Dukes)
Deveraux Octavian Basil (Mick Jagger and Melanie Hamrick)
Dimitri Portwood (Ashton Kutcher and Mila Kunis)
Dominic Michael (Rachael Finch and Michael Miziner)
Edward Alan Burrell (Alex Jones and Charlie Thomson)
Edward Aszard (Tatyana Ali and Vaughn Rasberry)
Eissa (Janet Jackson and Wissam Al Mana)
Elias (Michael Bublé and Luisana Lopilato)
Eli Christopher (Ellen Pompeo and Chris Ivery)
Enzo (Melissa and David Fumero)
Ernest ("Finn") Zhang (Cindy Halvorsen and Ernie Halvorsen)
Ernie William (Stephanie Izard and Gary Valentine)
Eros (Paulina Rubio and Gerardo Bazúa)
Eugene (Oscar Isaac and Elvira Lind)
Finley Jaiden (Jamie Vardy and Rebekah Vardy)
Flynn Maxwell (Patrick and Jasmin Renna)
Ford Douglas Armand (Armie Hammer and Elizabeth Chambers)
Forester Bruce Elijah (Elissa Reilly Slater and Brent Slater)
Forest Leonardo Antonio (Holly Madison and Pasquale Rotella)
Forest Sage Palmer (Teresa Palmer and Mark Webber)

# Baby Names

Forrest Henry (John and Candice Cody)
Freddie Reign (Louis Tomlinson and Briana Jungwirth)
Frederick Easton (Chris Klein and Laina Rose Thyfault)
Golden "Sagon" (Nick Cannon and Brittany Bell)
Grey Douglas (Molly Sims and Scott Stuber)
Greyson Valor (Jenni "JWoww" Farley and Roger Mathews)
Gunner Stone (Heidi Montag and Spencer Pratt)
Hal Auden (Benedict and Sophie Cumberbatch)
Hayden Joel (Ashley Jones and Joel Henricks)
Hemingway Nash (Benjamin Hollingsworth and Nila Hollingsworth)
Henry (Rachael Harris and Christian Hebel)
Henry Bear (Casey Wilson and David Caspe)
Henry Wilberforce (Jessa Duggar Seewald and Ben Seewald)
Hero (Terrence Howard and Mira Pak)
Hugo Wilson (Ginnifer Goodwin and Josh Dallas)
Hunter Zion (Jurnee Smollett-Bell and Josiah Bell)
Isaiah Sion Robert Nesta (David Nesta "Ziggy" Marley and Orly Marley)
Jack (Alexandra Breckenridge and Casey Neil Hooper)
Jack Clark (Annaleigh Ashford and Joe Tapper)
Jack Oscar (Rosie Huntington-Whitely and Jason Statham)
Jackson Kyle (Zach Roloff and Tori Roloff)
James Arthur IV (Brooke Anderson and Jim Walker)
James Miller (Ellie Kemper and Michael Koman)
Jameson Moon Hart (Pink and Carey Hart)
Jonathan Rosebanks (Anne Hathaway and Adam Schulman)
Joshua Bishop (Katherine Heigl and Josh Kelley)
Journey River (Megan Fox and Brian Austin Green)
Jru (Draya Michelle and Orlando Scandrick)
Jude (Jayma Mays and Adam Campbell)
Jude Daniel (Jaren and Evyn Mustoe Johnston)
Jude Malcolm (Steven Yeun and Joana Pak)
Kenzo (Kevin Hart and Eniko Parrish)

# Baby Names

Kingston (Lesley-Ann Brandt and Chris Payne Gilbert)
Kingston Saint (Katy Mison and Breaux Greer)
Kit Joseph (Wayne Rooney and Coleen Rooney)
Kodah Dash (Rod Dyrdek and Bryiana Dyrdek)
Lars Gerard (Mel Gibson and Rosalind Ross)
Lennox (and twin brother Phoenix) (Chris Bosh and Adrienne Bosh)
Lenon (and twin brother Leo) (Jaime Pressly and Hamzi Hijazi)
Lenyx Kai (Jeremy and Val Collins)
Leo (and twin brother Lenon) (Jaime Pressly and Hamzi Hijazi)
Levi Blaze (Sean Paul Henriques and Jodi "Jinx" Steward Henriques)
Levon (Charlotte Ronson and Nate Ruess)
Liam James (Lauren Conrad and William Tell)
Mack James (Allison Langdon and Michael Willessee, Jr.)
Mateo (and twin sister Eva Maria Dos Santos) (Cristiano Ronaldo)
Montague George Hector (Geri Halliwell/Ginger Spice and Christian Horner)
Noah Russell (Russell and Nina Westbrook)
Odie Sal (Ashley Williams and Neal Dodson)
Parker Emmanuel (Jess and Camille Carson)
Revel James Makai (Matthew Morrison and Renee Puente)
River Joe (Jeff Goldblum and Emilie Livingston)
River Jones (Paulina Gretzky and Dustin Johnson)
Robinson True (Samantha and Christian Ponder)
Ronan Laine (Megan Hilty and Brian Gallagher)
Samuel Scott (Derick Dillard and Jill Duggar Dillard)
Shai Aleksander (Peta Murgatroyd and Maksim Chmerkovskiy)
Sinan (Kendra Spears and Prince Rahim)
Sir (and twin sister Rumi) (Beyonce and Jay-Z)
Slate (Landon Donovan and Hannah Bartell)
Soltan (Asa Soltan Rahmati and Jermaine Jackson II)
Stefano Ercole Carolo (Pierre Casiraghi and Beatrice Borromeo)
Thomas South (Justin and Kate Moore)

# Baby Names

Valentine (Chris O'Dowd and Dawn O'Porter)
Watson Cole (Chelsea Houska and Cole Doboer)
William "Billy" (Jimmy Kimmel and Molly McNearney)
Wolfgang Xander (Matt Hardy and Rebecca Victoria Reyes-Hardy)
Zen (Zoe Saldana and Marco Perego)

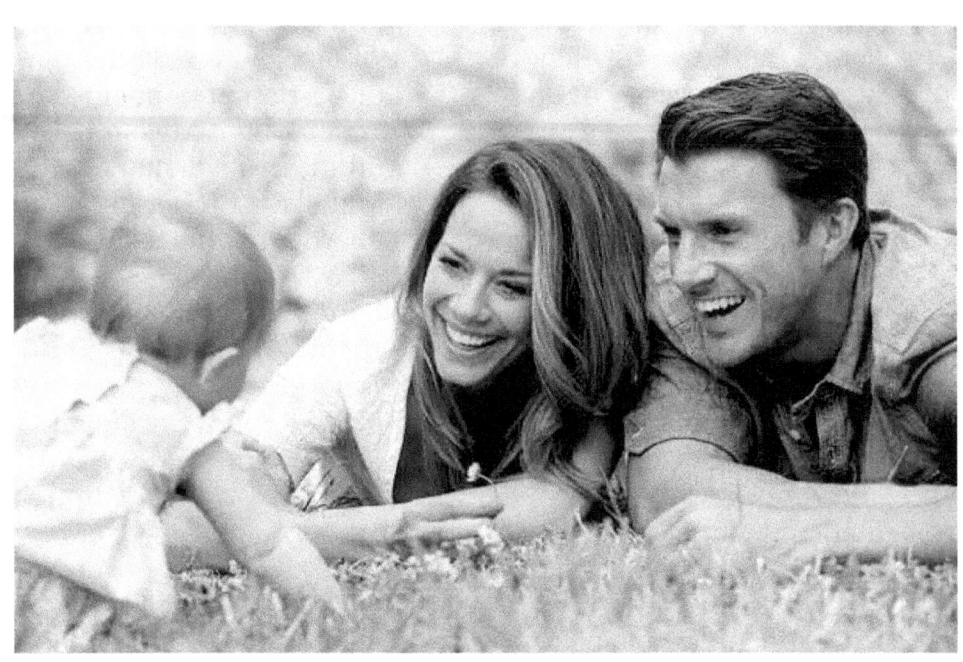

# Chapter 3: Impression Specific Names

**Strong boy names**
Brutus
Cerberus
Deimos
Gaston
Gunnar
Hades
Ivor
Jarek
Jarod
Poseidon
Rex
Salvador
Sigmund
Slade
Spartacus
Takashi
Timur
Trajan
Varg
Wolf

**Mature Boy names**
Adolfo
Agamemnon
Archibald
Arnold
Augustin
Aurelius
Constantin
Ernesto
Hannibal
Horatio
Ingram
Jehovah
Montgomery
Norbert Norman

Octavius
Spartacus
Steven
Ulysses
Vernon
Wolfram

**Strong girl names**
Boudicca
Bruna
Dagmar
Eoforhild
Gudrun
Hel
Hephzibah
Hilde
Hildegard
Jordana
Morag
Nemesis
Olga
Rebekka
Renate
Scheherazade
Sigrún
Storm
Tempest
Xena

**Mature girl names**
Agatha
Alfreda
Barbara
Drusilla
Eoforhild
Ester
Gertrude

# Baby Names

Griselda
Hera
Hildegard
Hortense
Juanita
Magorzata
Medusa
Mildred
Nemesis
Odelia
Olympia
Prudence
Theodor

**Wholesome boy names**
Benton
Cedar
Clarence
Edison
Eliot
Ernest
Franz
Freyr
Howard
Laurence
Leland
Leonard
Lincoln
Linden
Linus
Lionel
Moses
Paul
Steven
Wilbur

**Wholesome girl names**
Ann
Annmarie
Carol
Elowen
Emanuela
Emmaline
Essie
Fauna
Hilde
Honor
Lesley
Madelaine
Marigold
Marybeth
Marylou
Meadow
Nona
Rosemarie
Rosemary
Susan

**Smart boy names**
Aldous
Algernon
Astrophel
Charlemagne
Christoph
Clarence
Dilbert
Emrys
Franz
Freyr
Hermes
Montgomery
Mortimer
Neville
Octavius
Odysseus
Oswin
Sherlock
Steven

# Baby Names

Zephaniah

**Smart girl names**
Caterina
Eleonora
Emanuela
Freda
Freyja
Hermione
Hester
Hypatia
Ilse
Ione
Izabella
Lucrezia
Marceline
Małgorzata
Nemesis
Sappho
Silvana
Theodosia
Therese
Violetta

**Nature boy names**
Abraham
Arnie
Ben
Benjy
Cadfael
Cathal
Cedar
Charlie
Elia
Freyr
Lake
Liron
Llyr
Nathanael

Orrin
Quinlan
River
Robin
Steven
Tom
Uriah

**Nature Girl Names**
Autumn
Daisy
Fauna
Fawn
Fern
Ferne
Ffion
Hannelore
Hilde
June
Lavender
Lumi
Maryana
Meadow
Màiri
Natalya
Poppy
Rain
Rosemary
Spring

**Cunning boy names**
Abaddon
Adolph
Allah
Azazel
Bart
Beelzebub
Belial
Deimos

# Baby Names

Demon
Draco
Genghis
Israel
Judas
Lestat
Loki
Lucifer
Osama
Puck

**Cunning girl names**
Brandie
Gay
Gaynor
Gypsy
Hel
Jezebel
Lagina
Lakeisha
Latisha
Lilith
Medea
Medusa
Morana
Porsche
Roxy
Shaniqua
Skaði
Zarathustra

**Mysterious names**
Algernon
Azazel
Azriel
Belial
Castor
Cerberus
Deimos

Everard
Felicjan
Freyr
Hades
Icarus
Jupiter
Legolas
Mirza
Nero
Pegasus
Puck
Quetzalcoatl
Toirdhealbhach

**Mysterious girl names**
Ambrosia
Anemone
Bellatrix
Boudicca
Deja
Eartha
Eulalia
Idril
Jonquil
Kallistrate
Medea
Myfanwy
Nefertari
Nefertiti
Nemesis
Sappho
Scheherazade
Valkyrie
Zarathustra
Zlata
Zoraida

**Funny boy names**
Archie

# Baby Names

Arnie
Bart
Buddy
Buster
Chaz
Chip
Dada
Dũng
Flick
Hilarius
Iggy
Kirby
Mo
Pacey
Pip
Puck
Reggie
Steven
Willy

**Funny girl names**
Oral
Gay
Tit
Lagina
Latisha
Tiffani
Kiki
Jojo
Gaynor
Rainbow
Candy
Bee
Blondie
Trixie
Fergie
Kimmy
Randi
Candi

Gabby
Dolly

**Youthful boy names**
Iggy
Ryker
Kory
Timmy
Pip
Codie
Jace
Robby
Sonny
Flick
Spike
Richie
Frankie
Kip
Ryder
Kayden
Chip
Robbie
Junior

**Youthful girl names**
Abbi
Cherry
Honey
Kaycee
Kiki
Kimmy
Kyleigh
Livvy
Lulu
Lumi
Mandi
Miku
Miley
Scout

# Baby Names

Spring
Sunshine
Tiffani
Trixie
Usagi
Winnie

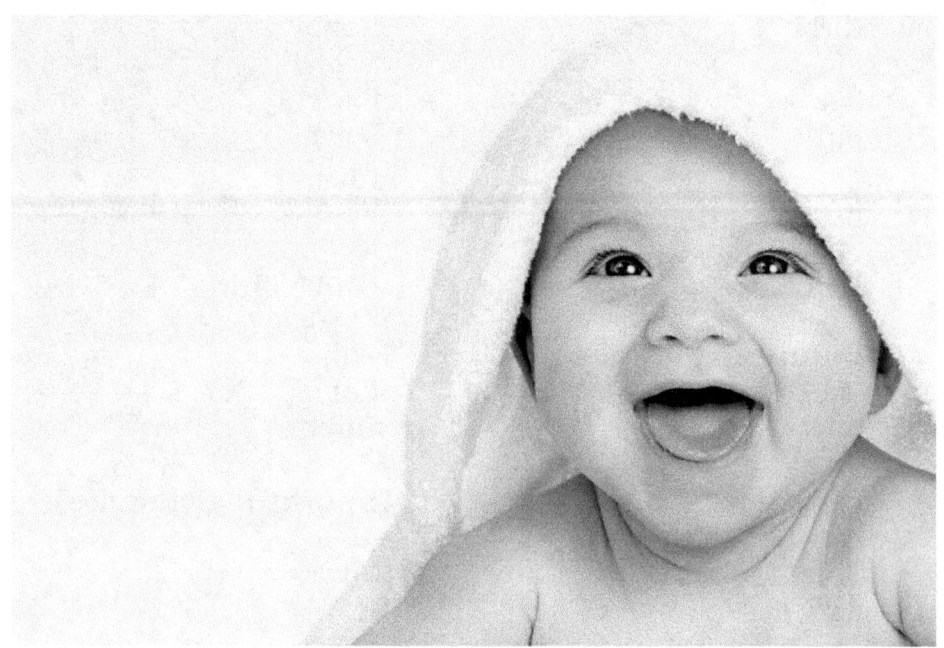

# Chapter 4: Biblical Baby Names

**Biblical Boy Names**

*Andrew:* The name Andrew has a Greek origin and means 'a strong man'.
Bible mention – Matt 4:18.

*Barak:* Barak means 'thunder' in Hebrew. Do not confuse it with Barack, which is an African name.
Bible mention – Judges 4:6.

*Daniel:* Daniel is a common biblical name for boys and means 'God is my judge'.
Bible mention – 1 Chron. 3:1.

*Ebenezer:* 'Rock of help' – with a meaning as strong as this, it is a pity that this Biblical boy name is not so popular.
Bible mention – 1 Sam. 4:1.

*Eliphaz:* Each life is a creation of God. Eliphaz means 'the endeavor of God'.
Bible mention – Gen. 36:4.

*Esau:* Esau means 'he who acts' in Hebrew. If you are looking for an uncommon Biblical baby boy names, try Esau.
Bible mention – Gen. 25:25.

*Ezekiel:* It may sound exotic but is a traditional Christian boy name. It means 'the strength of God' in Hebrew.
Bible mention – Ezekiel 1:3.

*Jairus:* In Hebrew, Jairus means 'my Light' or 'one who diffuses Light'.
Bible Mention – Mark 5:22.

*Jason:* Jason is a very popular biblical name but hasn't lost its charm. It means 'the one who cures'.
Bible mention – Acts 17:5

# Baby Names

*Micah:* Being humble is a virtue. Micah means 'humble' in Hebrew.
Bible mention – Judges 17:1.

*Matthias:* Matthias is a beautiful name and means 'the gift of the Lord'.
Bible mention – Acts 1:23.

*Nahum:* Another exotic name from the Bible! Nahum means 'comforter' in Hebrew.
Bible mention – Nahum 1:1

*Nadab:* The Hebrew language is full of beautiful names. Nadab means 'prince'.
Bible mention – Exodus 6:23.

*Omar:* The name Omar has its origin in both Hebrew and Arabic. It means 'he that speaks'.
Bible mention – Gen. 36:11.

*Obadiah:* Obadiah means 'the servant of the Lord'. It is a Hebrew name and is relatively uncommon.
Bible mention – 1 Kings 18:3.

*Othniel:* Here's a name that comes with a great nickname option – Niel! Othniel means 'the Lion of God'.
Bible mention – Joshua 15:17.

*Phineas:* For religious families, God is everything. If your family is the same, try Phineas to name your baby. It means 'the face of trust or protection'.
Bible mention – Exodus 6:25.

*Shadrach:* It is a relatively rare biblical name and means 'tender'.
Bible mention – Dan. 1:7.

*Titus:* Titus means 'pleasing' in Latin. It is a cute little name!
Bible mention – 2 Cor. 2:13.

# Baby Names

*Tobiah:* Another wonderful name from the Bible! Tobiah means 'Lord is good' in Hebrew.
Bible mention – Ezra 2:60.

*Uriah:* The meaning of the name Uriah is the very basis of any religion – faith. Uriah means 'the Lord is my light or fire'.
Bible mention – 2 Sam. 11:3

*Zebedee:* Zebedee means 'abundant' in Greek. Pay homage to God's abundant love for his children!
Bible mention – Matt. 4:21

*Elihu:* In Hebrew, Elihu means 'He is my God'. It is an unconventional name and will work for you if you are looking for a unique Christian name.
Bible mention – 1 Sam. 1:1

*Emmanuel:* It is a good choice for parents looking for traditional Christian names. It means 'God is with us' in Latin as well as Hebrew.
Bible mention – Isaiah 7:14

*Ethan:* The name Ethan comes from the Hebrew language and means 'strong'.
Bible mention – 1 Kings 4:31

*Isaac:* A common name, Isaac means 'laughter' in Hebrew.
Bible mention – Gen. 17:19

*Peter:* If you are looking for a name that has a universal appeal, nothing can beat the popularity of Peter. In Greek, it means 'a rock'.
Bible mention – Matt. 4:18

*Reuben:* Reuben means 'he who sees the Son' in Hebrew. Another gem from the Bible!
Bible mention – Gen. 29:32

# Baby Names

*Saul:* If you are looking for a beautiful name, with a great meaning, try Saul. It means 'the one who is in demand'.
Bible mention – 1 Sam. 9:2

*Shem:* Shem means 'renowned' in Hebrew. It will surely attract attention!
Bible mention – Gen. 5:32

*Abner:* The name Abner means 'the Father of Light' in Hebrew. It is a name that is rapidly climbing the popularity charts around the world.
Bible mention – 1 Sam. 14:50

*Abram:* Abram means 'exalted Father'. The name traces its origin to the Hebrew language.
Bible mention – Gen. 11:27

*Amaziah:* It screams fun but has a deep meaning. Amaziah means 'the strength of God' in Hebrew.
Bible mention – 2 Kings 12:21

*Aquila:* Are you looking for a Christian name that reflects your love for nature as well? How about Aquila? It means 'an eagle' in Latin.
Bible mention – Acts 18:2

*Asher:* Asher means 'happiness' in Hebrew and will hopefully help your child fill the world with love and laughter.
Bible mention – Gen. 30:13

*Malachi:* Does this name sound too exotic? But it is from the Bible! It means 'my messenger or angel' in Hebrew.
Bible mention – Mal. 1:1

*Michael:* Michael is the Latin word for 'humble'. It is an evergreen choice.
Bible mention – Num. 13:13

*Victor:* The Bible is all about the victory of good over evil. Victor means 'victory' in Latin.
Bible mention – 2 Timothy 2:5

*Zephaniah:* If you are game for a unique Christian name, consider Zephaniah. It means 'the Lord is my secret' in Hebrew.
Bible mention – 2 Kings 25:18

*Nathan:* Another popular name from the Bible, Nathan means 'rewarded' in Hebrew.
Bible mention – 2 Sam. 5:14

*Nehemiah:* Nehemiah means 'repentance of the Lord' in Hebrew. It is a great name for parents looking for a unique Christian name.
Bible mention – Neh. 1:1

*Noah:* Noah is an evergreen bible name for boys! It means 'consolation' in Hebrew.
Bible mention – Gen. 5:29

*Silas:* Is your son your third child? Try naming him Silas, which means 'third' in Latin.
Bible mention – Acts 15:22

**Biblical Girl Names**
*Atarah:* A beautiful name, Atarah means 'crown' in Hebrew. It is one of the perfect biblical girl names for your little princess. Bible mention – 1 Chron. 2:26

*Abigail:* Abigail means 'the father's joy'. Bible mention – 1 Sam. 25:3
Adriel: Here's one of the best Bible names for girls that is both religious and unique. Adriel means 'flock of God' in Hebrew. Bible mention – 1 Sam. 18:19

*Adah:* If you what you want is an uncommon name, from the Bible, go for Adah. It means 'an assembly' in Hebrew.

Bible mention – Gen. 4:19

*Bernice:* Bernice means 'one who brings victory' in Greek. It is a musical name and pretty traditional too.
Bible mention – Acts 25:13

*Bethany:* Bethany in Hebrew means 'house of song'. It is a very popular name!
Bible mention – Matt. 21:17

*Charity:* Charity is one of the beautiful Biblical names for girls that has its origin in the Latin language. It means 'dear'.
Bible mention – 1 Cor. 13:1-13

*Chloe:* A classic English name, Chloe means 'green herb' in Greek.
Bible mention – 1 Cor. 1:11

*Diana:* Yes, it is a beautiful name! It means 'luminous or perfect' in Latin.
Bible mention – Acts 19:27

*Elisha:* The Christian baby girl names grow elegant as we move. As pretty as a name can get, Elisha is a great choice for parents looking for a simple yet classy name. It means 'the Salvation of God' in Latin.
Bible mention – Luke 1:5

*Esther:* Nothing is more interesting than a little mystery. The Esther means 'secret or hidden' in Hebrew.
Bible mention – Esther 2:7

*Eva:* Short and sweet – Eva is the perfect name for families who like to keep things simple. It means 'living' in Hebrew.
Bible mention – Gen. 3:20

*Jael:* An uncommon yet interesting Christian name, Jael means 'one who ascends' in Hebrew.
Bible mention – Judges 4:17

# Baby Names

*Joanna:* If you want to give your daughter a name that is both Christian and trendy, you can consider Joanna. It means 'grace or gift of the Lord' in Hebrew.
Bible mention – Luke 8:3

*Julia:* If you are not averse to common names, you can give Julia a chance. It means 'soft and tender hair' in Latin. This christian girl baby names are common but popular.
Bible mention – Romans 16:15

*Jemimah:* The name Jemimah means 'as beautiful as the day' in Hebrew. If you want a name that is unique, try this beauty!
Bible mention – Job 42:14

*Joy:* Nothing can beat the beauty in simplicity. Joy – this simple word encompasses all that is good in the world. Joy means 'happiness' in Old French and Latin.
Bible mention – Heb. 1:9

*Mercy:* A beautiful name with an even more beautiful meaning! Mercy means 'compassion' in English.
Bible mention – Gen. 43:14

*Myra:* In Greek Myra means 'I flow'. This Christian girl names is poetic name and a favorite among parents who like modern yet classic names.
Bible mention – Acts 27:5

*Michal:* A name that means 'resembling God' just cannot go wrong! Michal is a Hebrew name.
Bible mention – 1 Sam. 18:20

*Miriam:* So, you thought Christian names are all about being docile? Think again! The very traditional sounding name Miriam means 'rebellion' in Hebrew.
Bible mention – Exodus 15:20

# Baby Names

*Olive:* Here's another Biblical name for baby girl, which is both traditional and popular. Olive means 'beauty or dignity' in Latin.
Bible mention – Gen. 8:11

*Ophrah:* Ophrah means 'fawn' in Hebrew. You can also use its more common spelling, Oprah.
Bible mention – Judges 6:11

*Paula:* The name means 'small or little' in Latin.
Bible mention – Acts 13:9

*Rachel:* Rachel means 'sheep' in Hebrew. The term sheep has deep relevance in the Bible. And if you are a fan of yesteryears hit sitcom, the name will have additional meaning.
Bible mention – Gen. 29:6

*Rebecca:* Rebecca was the wife of Isaac and the mother of Jacob and Esau. It is derived from a verb that means to be 'tied up' or 'beautifully ensnaring'. It also means 'soil'.
Bible mention – Gen. 24:14

*Ruth:* A very English name, Ruth means 'content' in Hebrew.
Bible mention – Ruth 1:4

*Sapphira:* An exotic name, Sapphira means 'that relates or tells' in English.
Bible mention – Acts 5:1

*Sarai:* Your daughter is your princess, right? Well, then give her a name that reflects just that! Sarai means 'my princess' in Hebrew.
Bible mention – Gen. 17:15

*Terah:* The name Terah means 'to blow or scent' in Hebrew. It is a great option for those looking for a unique Christian name.
Bible mention – Num. 33:27

Baby Names

*Tirzah:* Another gem of a name from the Bible! The name Tirzah means 'benevolent or pleasing' in Hebrew.
Bible mention – Numbers 26:33

*Tabitha:* Tabitha – a name straight out of storybooks! The beautiful name means 'a gazelle' in Aramaic.
Bible mention – Acts 9:36

*Victoria:* Some names never lose their charm. Victoria is one of them. It means 'victory' in Latin. If you like to give traditional names a modern twist, you can name your daughter Victory too.
Bible mention – Deut. 20:4

*Zemira:* Zemira has such a nice ring to it, don't you agree? It means 'a song' in Hebrew. This Christian name for girl is beautiful.
Bible mention – 1 Chron. 7:8

*Zina:* Zina is a Greek name that means 'shining'. It is an elegant name for your daughter.
Bible mention – 1 Chron. 23:10

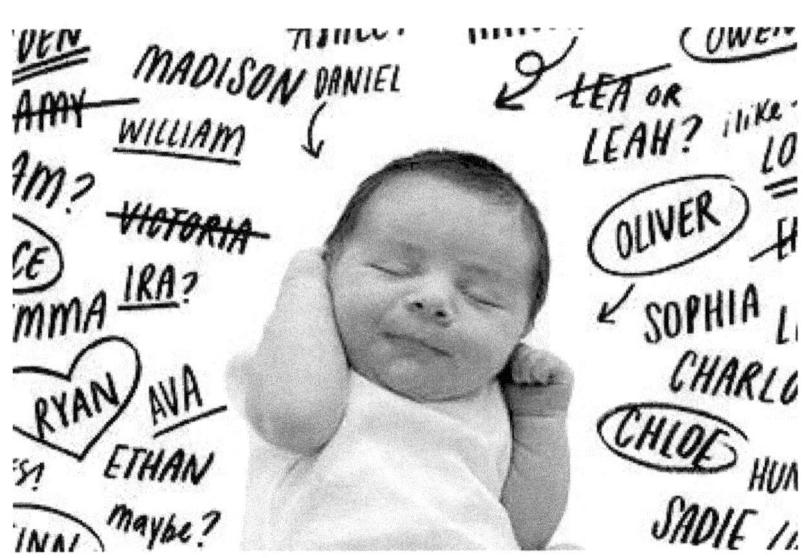

# Chapter 5: Unique Baby Names

**Cleverly spelled names**

Sometimes, all it takes to put a new spin on an old classic is a couple of extra letters. You can mix the vowels around, drop an extra Y in the middle, or change an existing Y to either eigh or ee. The ways you can modify existing names is practically endless, just don't get too carried away as otherwise you might end up with a name that no one can actually spell.

**Cleverly spelled girl names**
Abbagail
Arionna
Brystl
Brieanna
Cayli
Christal
Christean
Cloey
Emilee
Justise
Karleigh
Kassidy
Lynnsae
Madyson
McKenzie
Rashelle
Reanna
Shyann

**Cleverly spelled boy names**
Brayden
Carsyn
Cayden
Chantz
Damion
Dekan
Gavyn
Jaiden
Kameron
Landyn
Rian
Jaycee

## Unique, unexpected names
The class of 2036 will be sporting some names that may look a little odd now, luckily you have plenty of time to get used to them before they start popping up too regularly.

### Unique boy names
Angel
Anzen
Brantford
Camilo
Cayson
Callaghan
Coen
Corban
Cortez
Crew
Cyrus
Damari
Dangelo
Davon
Elian
Eliseo
Enoch
Ethen
Flynn
Gaige
Gibson
Haiden
Hayden
Ignacio
Jabari
Jakobe
Jaylon
Joziah
Kael
Keegan
Keon
Keyon
Kyan
Laken
Lathan
Leighton
Malaki
Mason
Maxton
Mustafa
Parker
Quinten
Raiden
Roderick
Sawyer
Thaddeus
Trace
Tre
Turner
Tyson
Vaughn
Vihaan
Yeggar
Yehuda
Zair

## Unique girls name

Addilyn
Adley
Analia
Armelle
Ashlynn
Aviana
Bexley
Brielle
Brinley
Britta
Bronwyn
Cadence
Calla
Camari
Ciara
Danica
Darby
Delaney
Dinah
Elora
Ember
Embry
Farren
Gracen
Grecia
Greer
Harlyn
Hartley

Hensley
Ina
Isa
Jaelyn
Kaia
Malena
Secora
Sephia
Shealyn
Tressa
Trinity

**Unique unisex names**

Adrian
Arron
Blaine
Blair
Brett
Carmen
Carson
Dallas
Dana
Drew
Elisha
Ellery
Emerson
Evan
Florian
Glen
Gracyn
Hadley
Hunter
Ira
Israel
Julian
Kelsey
Kendall
Lane
London
Marley
Mason
Michael
Montana
Nevada
Orion
Parker
Paxton
Peyton
Phoenix
Pressly
Quinn
Reese
Riley
Scout
Skye
Spencer
Tyler
Tyne
Wyatt
Wynne
Zane

## Names with interesting meanings

Texie (Derived from the name "Texas")
Cuba (Borrowed from the namesake island country)
Wava (Slavic name meaning "Stranger")
Ova (Latin word meaning "Egg")
Erie (Celtic name meaning "From Ireland")
Lavada (Old Scottish name meaning "High Place")
Almeta (Danish name meaning "Pearl")
Willodean (Unknown meaning, possibly a female variant of "Willard")
Jettie (Derived from name "Jetta")
Ferne (Derived from plant type "fern")
Alessia (Greek and Italian name meaning "Defender")
Anika (Hebrew name meaning "Grace")
Veola (From "Viola", Latin for "Flower")
Mika (Japanese name meaning "A New Moon")
Rasheeda (Arabic name meaning "Conscious, Pious, Wise, or Mature")
Theola (Greek name meaning "Divine")
Kelle (Gaelic name meaning "Slender, Fair")
Erminia (Feminine form of "Herminius", a Roman God)
Tamisha (Old American name meaning "Ram")
Roxy (Persian name meaning "Dawn, Bright")
Rhona (Welsh name meaning "Fair, Slender")
Ka (Egyptian name meaning "Spark of Life")
Amberly (Derived from color amber)
Jacinda (Greek name meaning "Beautiful")
Minda (Hindu name meaning "Light and Knowledge")
Roselle (Swedish name meaning "Rose")
Sharri (Hebrew name meaning "Plains")
Emerald (A type of deep green gemstone)
Arianne (Latin name from Ariadne, a mythical figure)
Lala (Hawaiian name meaning "Cheerful" or "Famous")
Blossom (English name meaning "Fresh")
Argelia (Latin name meaning "Full of Treasures")
Kenda (English name meaning "Child of Clear, Cool Water")

Avery (Old English name meaning "Elf" or "Counsel")
Valentine (Borrowed from St. Valentine)
Tory (English name meaning "From the Craggy Hills")
Viki (Latin name meaning "Conqueror")
Leena (Irish name meaning "Wed Meadow")
Maryland (Place name from namesake US state)
Eliz (Hebrew name meaning "God is My Oath")
Zetta (Hebrew name meaning "Olive")
Kendal (English name meaning "Valley of the River Kent")
Annelle (English variant of the Hebrew name Hannah, meaning "God Has Favored Me")
Divina (Latin name meaning "Divine One")
Keira (Gaelic name meaning "Dusky, Dark-Haired")
Maurita (Latin name meaning "Dark")
Buena (Spanish word meaning "Good")
Edra (Hebrew name meaning "Powerful")
Dakota (Native American name meaning "Friend")
Georgianne (Greek name meaning "Farmer", feminine form of "George")

# Chapter 6: Top 100 Baby Names

**Girls**

| | | | | |
|---|---|---|---|---|
| 1 | Sophia | | 36 | Kinsley |
| 2 | Olivia | | 37 | Hailey |
| 3 | Emma | | 38 | Madelyn |
| 4 | Ava | | 39 | Paisley |
| 5 | Isabella | | 40 | Elizabeth |
| 6 | Mia | | 41 | Addison |
| 7 | Aria | | 42 | Isabelle |
| 8 | Riley | | 43 | Anna |
| 9 | Zoe | | 44 | Sarah |
| 10 | Amelia | | 45 | Brooklyn |
| 11 | Layla | | 46 | Mackenzie |
| 12 | Charlotte | | 47 | Victoria |
| 13 | Aubrey | | 48 | Luna |
| 14 | Lily | | 49 | Penelope |
| 15 | Chloe | | 50 | Grace |
| 16 | Harper | | 51 | Elena |
| 17 | Evelyn | | 52 | Peyton |
| 18 | Adalyn | | 53 | Lillian |
| 19 | Emily | | 54 | Skyler |
| 20 | Abigail | | 55 | Natalie |
| 21 | Madison | | 56 | Charlie |
| 22 | Aaliyah | | 57 | Stella |
| 23 | Avery | | 58 | Savannah |
| 24 | Ella | | 59 | Kennedy |
| 25 | Scarlett | | 60 | Lila |
| 26 | Maya | | 61 | Liliana |
| 27 | Mila | | 62 | Bella |
| 28 | Nora | | 63 | Callie |
| 29 | Camilla | | 64 | Audrey |
| 30 | Arianna | | 65 | Lucy |
| 31 | Eliana | | 66 | Aurora |
| 32 | Hannah | | 67 | Hazel |
| 33 | Leah | | 68 | Makayla |
| 34 | Ellie | | 69 | Violet |
| 35 | Kaylee | | 70 | Reagan |

# Baby Names

| | |
|---|---|
| 71 | Emery |
| 72 | Emilia |
| 73 | Gabriella |
| 74 | Maria |
| 75 | Sophie |
| 76 | Claire |
| 77 | Everly |
| 78 | Allison |
| 79 | Eva |
| 80 | Eleanor |
| 81 | Melanie |
| 82 | Kylie |
| 83 | Nevaeh |
| 84 | Alice |
| 85 | Adeline |
| 86 | Alaina |
| 87 | Gianna |
| 88 | London |
| 89 | Naomi |
| 90 | Bailey |
| 91 | Serenity |
| 92 | Jocelyn |
| 93 | Juliana |
| 94 | Julia |
| 95 | Isla |
| 96 | Sadie |
| 97 | Ariel |
| 98 | Caroline |
| 99 | Jasmine |
| 100 | Clara |

**Interesting top girl name meanings**
- *Ada:* a name with plenty of feminist connotations set to be popular in 2018, meaning 'noble'.
- *Amelia:* a Greek name, meaning 'industrious'. Famous Amelias include flying legend Amelia Earhart, and two Princess Amelias of Great Britain during the eighteenth century.
- *Aurora:* A more unique Latin baby name, meaning 'dawn'.
- *Ava:* Latin, meaning 'like a bird'. Famous Avas' include Ava Gardner was an iconic American actress during the 1950s–1970s.
- *Ella:* a German baby name, meaning 'completely'. Now becoming a name in its own right, Ella is traditionally a shortened version of Eleanor, Elizabeth and Ellen.
- *Emily:* a Latin name, meaning 'rival, eager'. Emily Dickinson is one of the most well-known poets of the nineteenth century. A very popular name choice in recent years.
- *Emma:* Never far from the top of most popular baby name lists, Emma does not seem to be going anywhere yet. A traditional name meaning 'universal'.
- *Emmeline:* Another feminist name set to rise this year, an old French name meaning 'work'.
- *Evelyn:* Following the trend mentioned above, Evelyn looks set to be popular. A beautiful name meaning 'wished for child'.
- *Isabella:* 2018 is set to be a royal year, with a wedding and royal baby number three on the way. Isabella, a Spanish name meaning 'pledged to God' definitely has the royal seal of approval.
- *Isla:* a Scotish Gaelic baby name meaning 'river', set to be popular in 2018.
- *Ivy:* A botanical baby name that has risen in popularity since being chosen by Beyonce for her first child, Blue-Ivy.

# Baby Names

- *Jessica:* a Hebrew baby name, meaning 'He sees'. A popular name over several decades, cute alternatives include Jess and Jessie.
- *Luna:* A Latin baby name meaning 'moon' that has been rising in popularity over the past few years. A cute choice for Harry Potter fans!
- *Matilda:* In 2018, names that end in - a or have a - v sound will dominate for girls. One of our favourite, more unique baby names following this pattern is Matilda, meaning 'battle mighty'. Cute nicknames include Tilly.
- *Meghan:* With a royal wedding on the cards, this beautiful name is predicted to grow in popularity. Originally a Welsh name meaning 'pearl'.
- *Mia:* An Italian baby name meaning 'mine', set to rise in popularity this year.
- *Nora:* Following the trend in baby names ending with an -a sound, this cute choice is a traditional Irish baby name meaning 'light'.
- *Olivia:* a Latin name, meaning 'olive'. Olivia has featured in the Top 10 names for girls in England for several years now, including at number one.
- *Victoria:* Another royal baby name to celebrate a royal year, with an elegant feel to it, this traditional name means 'victory'.

**Boys**

| | | | | |
|---|---|---|---|---|
| 1 | Jackson | | 39 | Levi |
| 2 | Liam | | 40 | Cameron |
| 3 | Noah | | 41 | Nicholas |
| 4 | Aiden | | 42 | Josiah |
| 5 | Lucas | | 43 | Lincoln |
| 6 | Caden | | 44 | Dylan |
| 7 | Grayson | | 45 | Samuel |
| 8 | Mason | | 46 | John |
| 9 | Elijah | | 47 | Nathan |
| 10 | Logan | | 48 | Leo |
| 11 | Oliver | | 49 | David |
| 12 | Ethan | | 50 | Adam |
| 13 | Jayden | | 51 | Eli |
| 14 | Muhammad | | 52 | Landon |
| 15 | Carter | | 53 | Joseph |
| 16 | Michael | | 54 | Christian |
| 17 | Sebastian | | 55 | Ian |
| 18 | Alexander | | 56 | Anthony |
| 19 | Jacob | | 57 | Brayden |
| 20 | Benjamin | | 58 | Aaron |
| 21 | James | | 59 | Hunter |
| 22 | Ryan | | 60 | Adrian |
| 23 | Matthew | | 61 | Joshua |
| 24 | Daniel | | 62 | Andrew |
| 25 | Jayce | | 63 | Carson |
| 26 | Mateo | | 64 | Dominic |
| 27 | Caleb | | 65 | Asher |
| 28 | Luke | | 66 | Colton |
| 29 | Julian | | 67 | Christopher |
| 30 | Jack | | 68 | Jordan |
| 31 | William | | 69 | Bryson |
| 32 | Wyatt | | 70 | Ezra |
| 33 | Gabriel | | 71 | Easton |
| 34 | Connor | | 72 | Xavier |
| 35 | Henry | | 73 | Jeremiah |
| 36 | Isaiah | | 74 | Zane |
| 37 | Isaac | | 75 | Luca |
| 38 | Owen | | 76 | Charlie |

## Baby Names

| | |
|---|---|
| 77 | Nolan |
| 78 | Hudson |
| 79 | Damian |
| 80 | Thomas |
| 81 | Max |
| 82 | Evan |
| 83 | Jonathan |
| 84 | Miles |
| 85 | Elliot |
| 86 | Elias |
| 87 | Austin |
| 88 | Kai |
| 89 | Ezekiel |
| 90 | Xander |
| 91 | Maverick |
| 92 | Chase |
| 93 | Tristan |
| 94 | Jason |
| 95 | Cooper |
| 96 | Jameson |
| 97 | Gavin |
| 98 | Alex |
| 99 | Eric |
| 100 | Bentley |

Interesting top boy name meanings

- *Arthur:* Whilst there looks to be a spike in popularity for names that aren't technically human, such as Bear, if you're still looking for something more traditional, this cute baby name, meaning 'bear' has been around for years.
- *Atticus:* Meaning 'from Attica' this is a trendy name, popular with To Kill a Mockingbird fans.
- *Charlie:* Old German, meaning 'free man'. Popularised by Charles the Great (a.k.a. Charlemagne). Prince Charles is heir to the throne of England. Charles Dickens was one of the finest and most enduringly popular English authors.
- *Finn:* A lovely Irish baby name meaning 'fair or white' predicted to rise this year.
- *George:* Greek, meaning 'farmer'. Chosen by the Duke and Duchess of Cambridge for their son, born in July 2013, and third in line to the throne. If you're looking for something a little different, how about Giorgio?
- *Harry:* Old German, form of Henry, meaning 'home ruler'. Famous Harrys include Prince Harry, Harry Potter and One Direction singer Harry Styles.
- *Henry:* Old German, meaning 'home ruler'. There have been eight Kings of England named Henry, and in the unlikely event that Prince Harry found himself on the throne he would become Henry IX.
- *Jack:* From the Hebrew John, meaning 'God is gracious'. The UK's most popular boys' name for 14 years until fairly recently.
- *Jacob:* Hebrew, meaning 'he who supplants'. Ancestor of the tribes of Israel in the Bible. Cute nicknames include Jacob, Jaco and Jago.
- *Llyod:* First world war names look set to be popular again this year, so how about this cute baby name meaning 'grey'.
- *Logan:* Meaning 'small hollow' this traditional Scottish name is growing in popularity.

# Baby Names

- *Muhammed:* Arabic, meaning 'praiseworthy'. Acknowledged as the prophet and founder of Islam. The name is extremely popular in large parts of the world. British runner Mo Farah is the Olympic and world record holder for the 5,000 and 10,000 metres.
- *Noah:* Hebrew, meaning 'peaceful'. In the Bible, Noah is said to have built an ark to save two of every animal from a flood that covered the earth
- *Oliver:* Latin, meaning 'olive tree'. The UK's most popular boys' name in several recent years.
- *Reggie:* Sometimes, names that look or sound similar hang around for a while. In 2018, names that start with R- or Th- will be big winners for boys. We love Reggie, a cute name meaning 'counsel power'.
- *Reuben*: A Hebrew name meaning 'behold a son', another name set to be popular in 2018.
- *Theo:* A cool-sounding baby name meaning 'divine gift'. Names beginning with Th- are set to be popular for boys this year and this is a cute choice.
- *Thiago:* Pronounced 'chee-AH-go', this unique baby name means 'supplanter' and is set to rise this year.
- *Tom:* As we approach 2020 (can you believe it?), keep an eye out for names from the Roaring Twenties. Tom looks set to have a revival, a cute traditional name meaning 'twin'.
- *William:* Old German, meaning 'strong-willed warrior'. Famous Williams include Prince William, playwright William Shakespeare and rapper Will.i.am.

**Top unisex names**

1. Darcy
2. Devon
3. Liam
4. Sophia
5. Bayley
6. Ava
7. Jacob
8. William
9. Indiana
10. August
11. Parker
12. Daniel
13. Logan
14. Matthew
15. Abigail
16. Lucas
17. Jackson
18. Rowan
19. Davie
20. Oliver
21. Jayden
22. Alex
23. Gabriel
24. Samuel
25. Charlie
26. Joe
27. Harper
28. Dylan
29. Riley
30. Gray
31. Isaac
32. Jazz
33. Ashley
34. Elizabeth
35. Jaya
36. Wyatt
37. London
38. Owen
39. Evelyn
40. Caleb
41. Harper
42. Ryan
43. Jacky
44. Hunter
45. Levi
46. Jaxon
47. Flynn
48. Micah
49. Victoria
50. Isaiah
51. Thomas
52. Connor
53. Jeremiah
54. Lily
55. Josiah
56. Lillian
57. Logan
58. Reagan
59. Aria
60. Hero
61. Colton
62. Brooklyn
63. Brayden
64. Hudson
65. Jules
66. Phoenix
67. Evan
68. Jaden
69. Austin
70. Gavin
71. Nolan
72. Savannah
73. Adam
74. Chase

Baby Names

75. Kyle
76. Ian
77. Skylar
78. Cooper
79. Easton
80. River
81. Tyler
82. Asher
83. Mateo
84. Drew
85. Ellio
86. Aaliyah
87. Nico
88. Stella
89. Sadie
90. Carson
91. Mila
92. Gabriella
93. Kennedy
94. Hayden
95. Kaylee
96. Ezra
97. Bentley
98. Hazel
99. Sawyer
100. Kayden

# Chapter 7: Top Baby Names of 2018

**Trending names for girls in 2018**
Isabella breaks into the Top 10, (up 6 places to number 9), this year despite Isabelle with an 'e' falling two places to 24. David and Victoria Beckham's choice of girls' name, Harper is still storming up the charts too, six years after their daughter was born and is up 17 places to 22.

A new, edgy trend name, Willow is making its way up the charts rising 8 places to 25.

'Old lady' names are still popular too and this year it's old fashioned names like Ivy up 14 places to 21 closely followed by Elsie up 5 places to 31 and Maisie up 7 places to 42 that are captivating the imagination of new mums and dads.
New trends in girls' names?

Now ranked the third most popular name for baby girls in the UK, Islais a 'trend name' that has seen a show-stopping rise in the last decade. The name has crept its way up the charts from nowhere in 2000 to position 21 ten years later in 2010 to 16 in 2011 to 9 in 2012 and 7 in 2013, staying at position 4 since 2014 and this year hitting the number 3 spot. Other names that never even ranked in the top 100 back in 2000, are now making their mark, including Ava at 5, Sophiaat 8, Evie at 13, and Ruby currently at 23.

Other names breaking into the top 100 and showing a significant rise in popularity, include Iris which has broken into the Top 100, (up 6 places to 96), and Clara (up 10 places at 98). Hallie has also grown massively in popularity in the last year rising, 44 places to 86 and Aurora, the real name of Sleeping Beauty, is up 35 places and now at 82.

**On the decline**
Not all 'old lady' names are on the rise. The recently popular and edgy old lady name Esme is down 10 places to 36 and Eva is down 9 places to 37. Scarlett was once deemed a trend

name after finding fame thanks to the Four Weddings and a Funeral character is also set to decline in 2018 falling 7 places to 28.

Likewise, once a regular in the Top 10 for over a decade, Jessica is now down 6 places to 15 and Chloe, who was a consistent contender in the Top 10 ten for years is now down 6 places to 29.

Set to leave the top 100 in 2018 is Zoe which is down 11 places at 97 along with once popular Maddison down 15 places at 99. Megan too is just holding on in the Top 100 at 100th place but is down a dramatic 19 places from last year. Here is our full top 100 girls' names for 2018.

**Top 100 girl names for 2018**

| | | | | |
|---|---|---|---|---|
| 1 | Olivia - | | 24 | Isabelle down 2 |
| 2 | Amelia - | | 25 | Willow up 8 |
| 3 | Isla up 1 | | 26 | Phoebe down 1 |
| 4 | Emily down 1 | | 27 | Evelyn up 2 |
| 5 | Ava - | | 28 | Scarlett down 7 |
| 6 | Lily up 1 | | 29 | Chloe down 6 |
| 7 | Mia up 5 | | 30 | Florence down 3 |
| 8 | Sophia down 2 | | 31 | Elsie up 5 |
| 9 | Isabella up 6 | | 32 | Millie down 2 |
| 10 | Grace - | | 33 | Layla down 1 |
| 11 | Poppy up 2 | | 34 | Matilda down 3 |
| 12 | Ella down 4 | | 35 | Rosie up 2 |
| 13 | Evie down 2 | | 36 | Esme down 10 |
| 14 | Charlotte up 2 | | 37 | Eva down 9 |
| 15 | Jessica down 6 | | 38 | Lucy down 4 |
| 16 | Daisy up 3 | | 39 | Aria up 6 |
| 17 | Sophie down 3 | | 40 | Ellie down 2 |
| 18 | Freya down 1 | | 41 | Sofia up 2 |
| 19 | Alice up 1 | | 42 | Maisie up 7 |
| 20 | Sienna up 4 | | 43 | Erin down 2 |
| 21 | Ivy up 14 | | 44 | Lola down 4 |
| 22 | Harper up 17 | | 45 | Lilly up 2 |
| 23 | Ruby down 5 | | 46 | Thea up 2 |

# Baby Names

| | | | | |
|---|---|---|---|---|
| 47 | Imogen down 5 | | 84 | Darcey down 2 |
| 48 | Eliza up 3 | | 85 | Victoria up 11 |
| 49 | Bella up 6 | | 86 | Hallie up 44 |
| 50 | Molly - | | 87 | Martha up 4 |
| 51 | Hannah down 5 | | 88 | Amelie down 14 |
| 52 | Emma - | | 89 | Katie down 1 |
| 53 | Violet up 4 | | 90 | Bonnie up 17 |
| 54 | Luna up 31 | | 91 | Arabella up 8 |
| 55 | Amber down 2 | | 92 | Lacey down 14 |
| 56 | Lottie up 13 | | 93 | Annie - |
| 57 | Darcie up 6 | | 94 | Niamh - |
| 58 | Maya - | | 95 | Lyla - |
| 59 | Georgia down 5 | | 96 | Iris up 6 |
| 60 | Elizabeth down 4 | | 97 | Zoe down 11 |
| 61 | Zara up 15 | | 98 | Clara up 10 |
| 62 | Penelope up 5 | | 99 | Maddison down 15 |
| 63 | Holly down 19 | | 100 | Megan down 19 |
| 64 | Nancy down 2 | | | |
| 65 | Rose down 6 | | | |
| 66 | Emilia up 4 | | | |
| 67 | Harriet down 2 | | | |
| 68 | Gracie down 7 | | | |
| 69 | Darcy up 8 | | | |
| 70 | Mila up 9 | | | |
| 71 | Orla up 18 | | | |
| 72 | Abigail down 12 | | | |
| 73 | Jasmine down 7 | | | |
| 74 | Eleanor up 1 | | | |
| 75 | Anna down 11 | | | |
| 76 | Summer down 8 | | | |
| 77 | Robyn up 6 | | | |
| 78 | Lexi down 6 | | | |
| 79 | Heidi down 8 | | | |
| 80 | Annabelle down 7 | | | |
| 81 | Maria up 9 | | | |
| 82 | Aurora up 35 | | | |
| 83 | Leah up 4 | | | |

## Trending names for boys in 2018
Logan (up 7 places to 12) and Theo (up 7 places to 14) are set to break into the Top 10. Arthur and Reggie are also on the rise following the trend for 'old man' names with Arthur up 8 places to 23 and Reggie up 11 places to 35. Similarly, the names Alfie (no movement at number 8) and Archie (up 4 places to 13) are steadily making their way up the list in recent years.

## New trends in boys' names?
Jaxon is on the rise (up 6 places to 37) and is fast becoming a popular modern derivative of the eternally popular name, Jack. Another contemporary name on the rise and up 8 places into the Top 40 is Harley.

Interestingly, If we look back at the year 2000 there were a number of names that weren't even in the top 100 back then. Yet now they have a regular spot in the Top 20. This decade's trend names for boys include Theo now at 14, Archie at 13, Logan now 12th, Leo at 11, Oscar at 10, Freddie at 9 and Noah at number 5.

Names that have burst into the top 100 that could indicate early trends for the next decade include Hunter up 33 places to 69, Theodore up 23 places 70 and Grayson which broke into the Top 100 at 93 last year (up 37 places).

## On the decline
Once popular Joseph has moved down 6 places to 32 suggesting a drop in favour for traditional biblical names. Although fellow, modern biblical name Elijah is up 6 places to 39.

Also noting a decrease in popularity this year is Dylan down 9 places at 43 and Jake down 13 places at 48.

Set to lose their spots within the 2018 Top 100 is Jamie down 10 places at 94, Austin down 17 places at 97 and dropping out of the Top 100 in 2018 is the once hugely popular Ben who's holding on at 100th place but down 4 places on last year.

**Top 100 boy names for 2018**

1. Oliver -
2. Harry -
3. Jack -
4. George up 1
5. Noah up 2
6. Charlie down 2
7. Jacob down 1
8. Alfie -
9. Freddie up 1
10. Oscar down 1
11. Leo up 1
12. Logan up 7
13. Archie up 4
14. Theo up 7
15. Thomas down 2
16. James down 5
17. Joshua down 3
18. Henry down 2
19. William down 4
20. Max down 2
21. Lucas up 2
22. Ethan down 2
23. Arthur up 8
24. Mason down 2
25. Isaac -
26. Harrison down 2
27. Teddy up 6
28. Finley -
29. Daniel down 2
30. Riley -
31. Edward up 1
32. Joseph down 6
33. Alexander down 4
34. Adam up 3
35. Reggie up 11
36. Samuel -
37. Jaxon up 6
38. Sebastian up 3
39. Elijah up 6
40. Harley up 8
41. Toby down 2
42. Arlo up 18
43. Dylan down 9
44. Jude up 8
45. Benjamin down 7
46. Rory up 19
47. Tommy down 7
48. Jake down 13
49. Louie down 5
50. Carter up 17
51. Jenson down 1
52. Hugo up 10
53. Bobby up 21
54. Frankie up 4
55. Ollie down 13
56. Zachary down 7
57. David down 2
58. Albie up 21
59. Lewis down 3
60. Luca down 1
61. Ronnie up 8
62. Jackson down 15
63. Matthew down 9
64. Alex down 3
65. Harvey down 12
66. Reuben down 2
67. Jayden down 16
68. Caleb up 2
69. Hunter up 33
70. Theodore up 23

# Baby Names

71. Nathan down 5
72. Blake down 9
73. Luke down 16
74. Elliot down 2
75. Roman up 15
76. Stanley down 8
77. Dexter -
78. Michael down 3
79. Elliott up 3
80. Tyler down 9
81. Ryan down 8
82. Ellis up 3
83. Finn down 2
84. Albert up 10
85. Kai down 7
86. Liam up 5
87. Calum -
88. Louis down 12
89. Aaron down 6
90. Ezra up 8
91. Leon down 3
92. Connor down 6
93. Grayson up 37
94. Jamie down 10
95. Aiden down 6
96. Gabriel down 4
97. Austin down 17
98. Lincoln up 24
99. Eli up 5
100. Ben down 4

**Top gender-neutral baby names for 2018:**
These are definitely hot stuff right now and are predicted to be big winners in the coming years as parents move toward more fluid notions of gender and identity.

*Max:* A Latin baby name meaning greatest. It's been popular for boys for years but is now being used as a girl's name too.

*Alex:* A cute, gender neutral baby name meaning 'defending men'.

*Charlie:* Meaning 'free man', for years this has been a diminutive of Charles or Charlotte.

*Andy:* Traditionally a shortened version of the name 'Andrew', this is now becoming a more popular choice for both sexes.

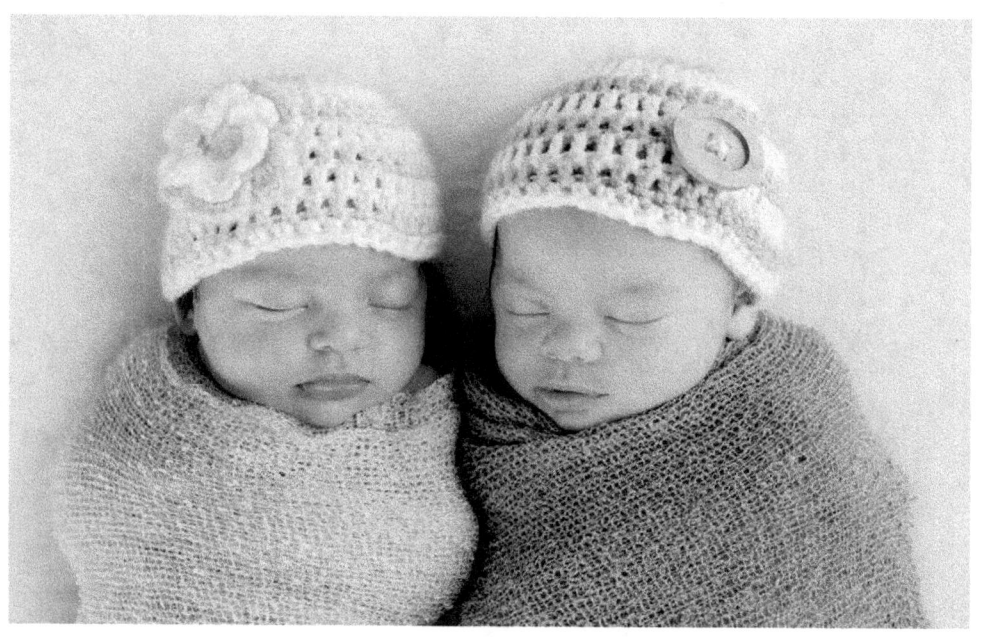

# Chapter 8: Traditional Baby Names

While a modern name can help you to jump on to an emerging trend and a trendy name might help you tap into the current cultural zeitgeist, there is an argument to be made for traditional names for a reason. These names became classics for a reason, take a look and you are sure to see some of your favorites.

**Traditional Girl Names**

- Alexa
- Allison
- Anastasia
- Anna
- Annelies
- Annelise
- Annika
- Antonia
- Arden
- Ashley
- Astrid
- Athena
- Beatrice
- Bridget
- Chloe
- Constanza
- Cosima
- Cynthia
- Eliska
- Eliza
- Elsa
- Frida
- Gisela
- Grace
- Greta
- Hannah
- Helena
- Honor
- Imogen
- Ingrid
- Jasmine
- Johanna
- Josephine
- Josie
- Juliet
- Katie
- Kirsten
- Lara
- Laurel
- Lauren
- Leonora
- Linnea
- Lydia
- Madeleine
- Phoebe
- Polly
- Rachel
- Rebecca
- Romy
- Rosa
- Rosalind
- Rowena
- Samantha
- Sandra
- Serena
- Sophia
- Theodora

**Traditional Boy Names**

Aaron
Abraham
Adam
Alden
Andrew
Asa
Augustus
Benjamin
Benton
Brooks
Christopher
Cyrus
Daniel
David
Davis
Dominick
Elliott
Emanuel
Emerson
Emilio
Grady
Hugo
Israel
Ivan
James
Jason
Jasper
Jefferson
Jeffrey
John
Joshua
Julian
Kevin
Lorenzo
Lucas
Major
Mark
Matthew
Max
Miles
Miller
Nathan
Nicholas
Noel
Oliver
Preston
Prince
Rafael
Raphael
Reed
Robert
Rocco
Samuel
Scott
Simon
Theo
Thomas
Timothy

**Traditional Unisex Names**
Ainsley
Augustine
Brodie
Camille
Claude
Dallas
Dominique
Ennis
Glenn
Hilary
Indra
Jade
Jody
Kim
Lindsay
Maxime
Morgan
Paris
Quinn
Robin
Sasha
Sean
Shannon
Shawn
Sidney
Sydney
Taylor
Terry
Tully
Yael
Yannick

## New spellings of traditional names

*Olivia/Alivia* – This name that means "olive tree" is given a more modern spin when starting with -a rather than the more traditional -o.

*Mia/Maya* – This name that means "water" is a beautiful Hebrew feminine name. And if pronounced with a long -i, it can also be spelled "Maya."

*Max/Macks* – A name that means "greatest," Max been popular for decades. Changing the -x to -cks gives it more of a modern touch.

*John/Jon* – John is a traditional name that means "God is gracious." It gets a more contemporary spin by dropping the -h.

*Devon/Devyn* – A gender neutral name that has substituted the -y for a modern version.

*Zoe/Zoey* – This name that means "life" is commonly seen spelled both ways.

*Aubrey/Aubree* – A popular name that means "elf ruler," Aubrey has appeared in the top 10 baby names — and updated with the -ee, has soared in popularity.

*Emily/Emilee* – The name that means "rival" is reinvented with a trendy -ee on the end.

*Jackson/Jaxon* – Adding the x has been popular with parents and has brought that spelling of the name up into the top 50 most popular baby names. Meaning "son of Jack," it is now more commonly spelled with the -x.

*Caitlin/Kaytlynn* – This traditional name that means "pure" is Irish and Welsh. Adding the alternative spelling gives it a more modernized spin.

*Rebecca/Rebekah* – The name that means "servant of God" is seen throughout the Bible spelled with a -k.

*Jane/Jayne* – Adding a -y to this popular name that means "God's gracious gift" adds a modern touch to a name that's not so plain.

*Amy/Aimee* – The name that means "beloved" has always been popular — and we love the French spelling of the name, Aimee.

*Jacob/Jakob* – A biblical name meaning "supplanter," this name has been popular with the traditional spelling for many years. If you want to update the traditional name, swap the -c for a -k.

*Sophia/Sofia* – You can't go wrong with this feminine name that means "wisdom." However you decide to spell it, we know it's a name that will grab attention.

*Catherine/Kathryn* – There are various ways to spell this popular and traditional name that means "pure."

# Chapter 9: Additional Baby Names A-Z

**Girls**

Abby
Adaline
Adalyn
Adalynn
Adelaide
Adelyn
Adriana
Alaina
Alana
Alani
Alayna
Alexa
Alexandra
Alexandria
Alexis
Alina
Alivia
Aliyah
Allison
Alyssa
Amara
Amaya
Amina
Amiyah
Ana
Anastasia
Andrea
Aneesah
Angel
Aniyah
Annabelle
Anzani
Arabella
Ariel
Ariella
Ashley

Athena
Avah
Ayla
Bailey
Blake
Blakely
Brianna
Brinley
Brooke
Brooklynn
Callie
Catalina
Charlie
Daisy
Dakota
Delilah
Destiny
Diana
Eden
Elaina
Elise
Eliza
Elliana
Eloise
Ember
Emberson
Emerson
Emersyn
Evelynn
Everleigh
Evie
Faith
Finley
Fiona
Freya
Gabrielle

Baby Names

| | |
|---|---|
| Genesis | Kimberly |
| Genevieve | Kylie |
| Georgia | Laila |
| Gia | Laura |
| Gracie | Lauren |
| Hadley | Leia |
| Harley | Leila |
| Harmony | Leilani |
| Heaven | Lexi |
| Helena | Lia |
| Hope | Lila |
| Iris | Liliana |
| Isabel | Lilly |
| Isla | Little |
| Ivy | Logan |
| Jade | Lola |
| Jasmine | London |
| Jhazelle | Londyn |
| Jocelyn | Loreli |
| Jordyn | Lydia |
| Josephine | Lyla |
| Josie | Madeline |
| Journee | Maggie |
| Journey | Makayla |
| Joy | Malia |
| Juliana | Mariah |
| Julianna | Mariam |
| Juliet | Marley |
| Juliette | Maryam |
| June | Mayli |
| Kaia | Mckenzie |
| Kali | Melanie |
| Kamila | Melody |
| Kate | Michelle |
| Katherine | Molly |
| Kayla | Morgan |
| Kendall | Mya |
| Khloe | Naliah |
| Kiara | Natalia |

# Baby Names

Nicole
Nina
Noelle
Norah
Nyla
Olive
Paige
Paislee
Paris
Parker
Payton
Presley
Princess
Raegan
Raelyn
Raelynn
Reabetsoe
Reagan
Rebecca
Reese
Remi
River
Rosalie
Rose
Rowan
Royalty
Ruby
Ryan
Ryleigh
Sage
Samantha
Sara
Sawyer
Selena
Serena
Sienna
Sydney
Taylor
Teagan

Thea
Trinity
Valentina
Valeria
Valerie
Vera
Vivian
Vivienne
Ximena
Zara
Zuri

**Boys**
Abel
Abraham
Ace
Adriel
Ahmad
Ahmere
Aidan
Aj
Alan
Alejandro
Ali
Amari
Amelia
Amir
Andres
Angel
Antonio
Arthur
Ashton
August
Austin
Axel
Ayaan
Basha
Beau
Ben
Bennett
Bentley
Blake
Bradley
Brandon
Brantley
Braxton
Brody
Brooks
Bryan
Bryce
Caden

Caiden
Calvin
Camden
Carlos
Cayden
Charles
Chase
Cole
Collin
Colt
Conner
Conor
Cruze
Damian
Damien
Dawson
Dean
Declan
Diego
Elliot
Elliott
Emerson
Emiliano
Emmanuel
Emmett
Enzo
Eric
Everett
Felix
Finn
Gael
George
Giovanni
Graham
Grant
Harper
Harrison
Hayden
Holden

# Baby Names

| | |
|---|---|
| Ibrahim | Luis |
| Israel | Lukas |
| Ivan | Maddox |
| Jaden | Madison |
| Jaiden | Malachi |
| Jake | Marcus |
| Jameson | Mark |
| Jasper | Matias |
| Jax | Matteo |
| Jay | Maximus |
| Jayce | Maxwell |
| Jesse | Messiah |
| Jesus | Miguel |
| Jobie | Miles |
| Joel | Milo |
| Jonah | Mohammad |
| Jose | Mohammed |
| Juan | Myles |
| Jude | Nathaniel |
| Junior | Nicolas |
| Justin | Olivia |
| Kaden | Omar |
| Kaiden | Oscar |
| Kaleb | Parker |
| Karson | Patrick |
| Karter | Paul |
| Kenneth | Paxton |
| Kevin | Peyton |
| Killian | Phoenix |
| Knox | Preston |
| Kyle | Prince |
| Kyrie | Quinn |
| Lane | Rafael |
| Leon | Remington |
| Leonardo | Rhett |
| Little | Richard |
| Lorenzo | Riley |
| Louis | River |
| Luca | Robert |

# Baby Names

Romeo
Rowan
Ryder
Ryker
Sam
Sean
Silas
Sophia
Steven
Theo
Theodore
Thiago
Timothy
Tristan
Troy
Tucker
Tyler
Victor
Vincent
Waylon
Wesley
Weston
Xander
Zachary
Zander
Zane
Zayden
Zayn
Zion

# Conclusion

Thank you for making it through to the end of *Baby Names*, let's hope it was informative and able to provide you with all of the tools you need to find the perfect baby name for your new baby. With so many names running through your head at the moment, it may seem as though this book has done more harm than good, providing you with countless options that you had not previously considered. While you may not be able to come to any concrete conclusions at the moment, if you put this book down and give yourself some time to think, you will likely find a number of names that you can't get out of your mind.

If you find that the idea of the literal timeclock on the decision is making it impossible for you to make a final choice, then what you really need to do is to stop and take a deep breath. While names are typically decided upon before the child is born, it is perfectly acceptable to wait a while before landing on the perfect name. Your child isn't going to be responding to anything, anytime soon so you have some time if you just can't seem to get it right.

Above all else, it is important to not get so worked up over making the decision that you fail to actually make a decision. With all the possibilities out there, it can be difficult to truly narrow it down, but if you fail to do so then you will ultimately be no better off than when you started. Instead, it is better to bite the bullet and make a choice in one direction or another. Even if you are unsure of the name you ultimately chose at first, with a little bit of time, you will likely find that it suits your child so well that you would be hard-pressed to come up with something better.

Finally, if you found this book useful in any way, a review on Amazon is always appreciated!

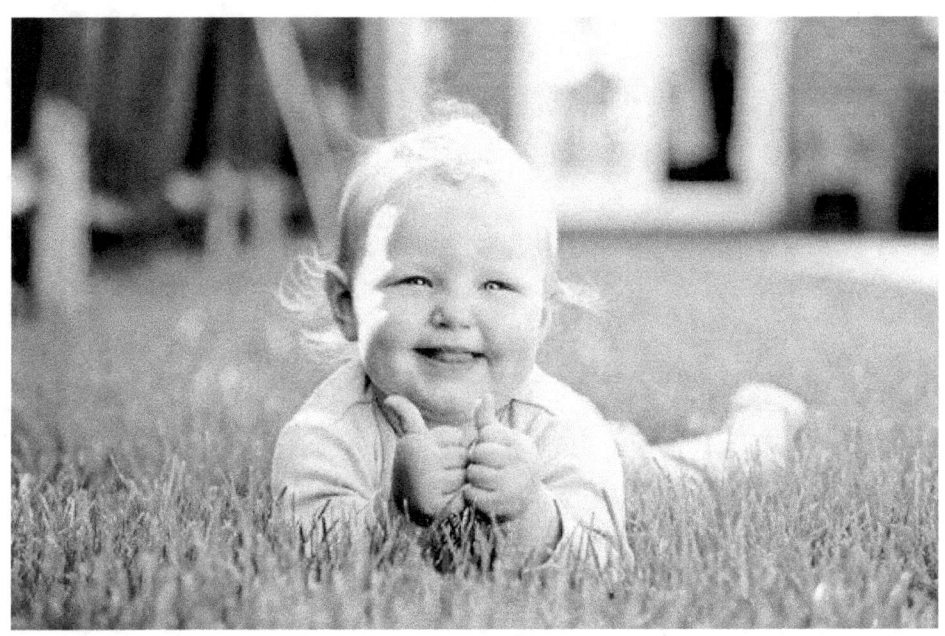

www.ingramcontent.com/pod-product-compliance
Lightning Source LLC
Chambersburg PA
CBHW072108290426
44110CB00014B/1866